Supporting the Development of a Vision and Strategic Plan for Zhejiang University's Academic Medical Center

Rafiq Dossani, Peggy G. Chen, Christopher Nelson

Sponsored by Zhejiang University

For more information on this publication, visit www.rand.org/t/RR2819

Library of Congress Cataloging-in-Publication Data is available for this publication

ISBN: 978-1-9774-0196-0

Published by the RAND Corporation, Santa Monica, Calif.

© Copyright 2019 RAND Corporation

RAND® is a registered trademark.

Cover image courtesy Zhejiang University

Support RAND

Make a tax-deductible charitable contribution at
www.rand.org/giving/contribute

www.rand.org

Preface

Zhejiang University is developing an academic medical center (AMC) in Hangzhou. The Center, which is under construction as of the writing of this report in late 2018, aims to undertake research and training and to provide clinical care in a collaborative and integrated environment. As this is the first time that these activities will be provided in an integrated way within Zhejiang University, the RAND Corporation was asked to recommend ways of organizing the AMC's activities to support its goals.

This report identifies and assesses potential models of organization to help achieve the goals of Zhejiang University's AMC. The study was performed by RAND Health Care and RAND Education and Labor for Zhejiang University.

RAND Health Care, a division of the RAND Corporation, promotes healthier societies by improving health care systems in the United States and other countries. We do this by providing health care decisionmakers, practitioners, and consumers with actionable, rigorous, objective evidence to support their most complex decisions. For more information, see www.rand.org/health-care.

RAND Education and Labor, a division of the RAND Corporation, conducts research on early childhood through postsecondary education programs, workforce development, and programs and policies affecting workers, entrepreneurship, financial literacy, and decisionmaking. Questions about this report should be directed to rdossani@rand.org, and questions about RAND Education and Labor should be directed to educationandlabor@rand.org.

Contents

Figures and Tables

Figures

Tables

Summary

Zhejiang University (ZJU) is a nationally ranked (top five) comprehensive university in China, with strengths in earth sciences, natural sciences, applied sciences, information sciences, medicine, and engineering. Its health care–related faculties include a School of Medicine, a School of Public Health, and a College of Pharmaceutical Sciences. The university has eight affiliated hospitals, both general and specialized, many of which are nationally ranked among the best in their fields. The university, the Yuhang District Government, and donors have invested resources for the development of ZJU's academic medical center (AMC) at a newly built campus in the Yuhang District. The AMC intends to integrate the university's health-related research, teaching, and care activities; build world-class comprehensive biomedical and clinical research infrastructure to provide vital patient care; support public health initiatives; conduct cutting-edge biomedical and clinical research; and educate the country's future health care workforce.

The AMC aims to accomplish these goals through the creation of an enabling environment with critical research support facilities and governing bodies that enhance collaborative learning; incorporation of global standards on clinical trials and human subject protections; innovation-driven expansion of the knowledge frontier in national and global health care; and sustainability of manpower, physical infrastructure, and finances. The AMC environment strives to have university-wide, national, and global effects.

The purpose of this study was to provide advisory support for the AMC. In particular, RAND researchers were asked to identify and assess potential models of organization that could help the ZJU AMC achieve its goals.

Building on an exercise that was started in early 2018 by ZJU's School of Medicine, we identified the following key domains of AMC organizational structure that have the potential to distinguish AMCs from one another: ownership and identity, governance and operations, and finances. We then conducted a review of four leading U.S.-based AMCs to understand how they differ in these domains. We reviewed available published evidence and held discussions with key informants of these AMCs to determine how their models might be applied to ZJU, and to better identify specific factors that might be appropriate for adoption. Beyond simply understanding the features of the various systems, we sought to understand how adoption of a specific model might function given the characteristics and goals of the ZJU AMC. We also dedicated time during discussions to elicit discussants' views of strengths and gaps in their own organization and governance system and, where possible, to understand how these models came into existence. The case study findings were discussed with policy-makers at ZJU to obtain their feedback and to refine RAND's work on organizational structure development.

Although potential models of organization could lie anywhere on the spectrum of the identified domains of the AMC organizational structure, based on our understanding of ZJU characteristics and goals, we identified four models with variations in these domains that ZJU could reasonably consider for governance of the new AMC. In all four models, ownership is divided between the university and the hospital (while governance is shared), but the models differ in where their identity lies and who holds operational control. We then reviewed the strengths and weaknesses of each of the four models and rated their potential in helping to meet the goals of the ZJU AMC. Based on our assessment, the following are our recommendations for ZJU, ranked in order of highest to lowest performance ratings.

1. **A university-led model**, in which the AMC adopts the identity of the university and is operated by the university.
2. **An autonomous model (or AMC-led model)**, in which the AMC adopts the identity of the university but operates independently.
3. **A hospital-led model**, in which the AMC adopts the identity of the hospital and is operated by the hospital.
4. **A shared model**, in which the AMC adopts the identity of the university and is operated jointly by the hospital and the university.

Each model brings advantages and challenges in addressing the goals of the ZJU AMC. Establishing a new system also comes with its own challenges that will need to be addressed.

Finally, we note that no matter which governance model is ultimately selected, there are likely to be unanticipated barriers that will require adjustments to the model even as progress continues. Thus, it is important that all aspects of design and implementation be informed by ongoing monitoring and evaluation. Together these factors will ensure the presence of learning and feedback loops that can guide ZJU in making midcourse corrections.

Acknowledgments

The authors would like to thank Zhengping Xu and his colleagues at the Zhejiang University Medical System. The authors would also like to thank the interviewees at Harvard Medical School, Stanford Medicine, University of California, Los Angeles Health, and University of Washington Medicine. Maria Vega provided expert editorial and communication support. We thank the reviewers, Jennifer Bouey and Ramya Chari.

Abbreviations

AMC	academic medical center
AMC-H	academic medical center–hospital division
AMC-R	academic medical center–research division
AMC-S	academic medical center–school of medicine division
BOT	board of trustees
CEO	chief executive officer
CMO	chief medical officer
CPS	College of Pharmaceutical Sciences
DGSOM	David Geffen School of Medicine
EC	executive committee
HMS	Harvard Medical School
IRB	institutional review board
MBBS	Bachelor of Medicine and Bachelor of Surgery
MD	Doctor of Medicine
MS	Master of Science
NIH	National Institutes of Health
Ph.D.	Doctor of Philosophy
RRMC	Ronald Reagan Medical Center
SOM	School of Medicine

SPH	School of Public Health
UCLA	University of California, Los Angeles
UW	University of Washington
ZJU	Zhejiang University

CHAPTER ONE

Background and Objectives

Introduction

Zhejiang University (ZJU) is a nationally ranked (in the top five) comprehensive university in China, with strengths in earth sciences, natural sciences, applied sciences, information sciences, medicine, and engineering. Its health care faculties include a School of Medicine (SOM), a School of Public Health (SPH), and a College of Pharmaceutical Sciences (CPS).

The SOM has eight affiliated hospitals, both general and specialized, many of which are nationally ranked among the best in their fields. The SOM has 600 faculty members and more than 6,000 students. The affiliated hospitals are legally independent entities, and together they host 12,000 beds and have a staff of more than 20,000. They are connected to ZJU's SOM by a contract of affiliation that assigns the SOM with the roles of representing ZJU and providing oversight to the academic linkages between the university and the affiliated hospitals. This includes components of training of students for the Doctor of Medicine (MD), Master of Science (MS), and Doctor of Philosophy (Ph.D.) programs; translational and clinical research, including interdisciplinary components; and research-oriented clinical care.[1]

China has an urgent need for better research, practice, and teaching in health care. The national government has announced a Double First Class initiative,[2] which aims to build world-class universities and first-class academic specialties throughout China. It has identified certain public universities, including ZJU, that will receive support to implement innovative approaches.

In response to this initiative, ZJU has promoted three major plans relating to health and health care:

---

[1] The SOM offers both the traditional five-year Bachelor of Medicine and Bachelor of Surgery (MBBS) and U.S.-style MD programs, which last for eight years. The use of "MD" here is intended to signify both the MBBS and MD programs.

[2] Australian Government, Department of Education and Training, "Implementation Measures Released for China's New-World Class University Policy," January 2017.

- Forming clinical innovation centers within hospitals.
- Establishing the Institute of Translational Medicine.
- Building a research-oriented Academic Medical Center (AMC) to promote cross-disciplinary research and development in medicine.

There are currently three clinical innovation centers in general hospitals affiliated with ZJU. The Institute of Translational Medicine was opened in 2014. The AMC, as of late 2018, is under construction.

The AMC at ZJU

An *Academic Medical Center* is defined as an organization that integrates and "aligns the education of health care professionals, biomedical research, and patient care/population health."[3] It usually includes an SOM along with other relevant professional schools (e.g., nursing, public health, pharmaceutical sciences), coupled with one or more hospitals or other patient-care entities. The term is intended to encompass all the health care activities of a university and its clinical care affiliates and assumes a high level of integration between them. Through such integrated work, an AMC provides vital clinical care, supports public health initiatives, conducts cutting-edge research, and educates the future health care workforce. This structure inherently involves the need for communication, collaboration, and possible compromise between member entities. The need for enhanced collaboration and communication is also key given the desire of member entities to foster innovation and bench-to-bedside translation of research through multidisciplinary research and development.

The AMC at ZJU, as currently envisaged, is a narrower concept. Instead of encompassing all health care–related activities, it is a newly proposed component of the existing medical system at ZJU; the latter consists of an affiliated group of institutions that includes an SOM, a SPH, a CPS, and eight hospitals. All the hospitals are legally independent entities.

Known also as the "Medical Center," the proposed AMC aims to contain a research module and a clinical module. The research module will be managed by the SOM and will focus on clinical, translational, and interdisciplinary research. The clinical module will focus on clinical care (patient care) and will be managed by one of ZJU's affiliated hospitals, First Affiliated Hospital (a comprehensive hospital). By con-

---

[3]   Association of Academic Health Centers, "Academic Health Centers: Leading Healthcare Transformation," webpage, undated. Non-core processes that might be integrated include consolidation of administrative research services, such as reference services, institutional review board (IRB) processes, ethics training, information technology systems, and grants and contracts management. Core processes that could be integrated include consolidating staff appointment, staff development, and staff promotion processes.

trast, at present, biomedical research takes place within the SOM, and clinical research occurs in the hospitals.

Ownership of the physical infrastructure will be divided between the university, which will own the research facilities, and First Affiliated Hospital, which will own the clinical facilities. However, the intent is to closely link the two research and clinical modules through the academic components of training students for MD, MS, and Ph.D. programs, translational and clinical research, including interdisciplinary components; and research-oriented clinical care.[4] The AMC has also received the support of the local government (Yuhang District Government of Hangzhou City). Technology firm Alibaba has donated 560 million renminbi to the clinical module.

ZJU's aspiration is that the Medical Center, despite its narrow role, will still fulfill the functions of an all-encompassing AMC (i.e., provide vital clinical care, conduct cutting-edge research, and educate the nation's future health care workforce). All of these activities will overlap with activities occurring elsewhere in the ZJU Medical System. Some of the overlaps will merely continue existing overlaps (e.g., the eight hospitals within the system already provide many overlapping clinical services and undertake overlapping clinical research). Other overlaps will be new, with potentially significant and unexplored consequences (e.g., establishing some education and basic science and translational research services in the AMC while continuing with some of these services at the SOM).

The proposed AMC will undoubtedly face challenges, including building staff commitment to an integrated entity with the various accompanying commitments of resource sharing and functioning under a new organizational structure and its potentially new governance mechanisms.

Goals of the ZJU AMC and the Need for a Stronger Organizational Structure

ZJU has identified the following goals for the ZJU AMC:

- innovative research, training, and care, encompassing medical care, education, and research
- quality of research, training, and care comparable with global best practices
- sustainability of manpower, physical infrastructure, and financial resources
- compliance with local laws, regulations, and capacity constraints.

---

[4]   ZJU's focus is on integrating the SOM with the hospitals within the AMC structure. The other schools will be integrated later. Therefore, in this report, we do not consider how the CPS and the SPH will be integrated into the AMC.

The AMC should be more than just "one more" component of ZJU's health care system. Rather, it should house and develop the best talents of the SOM, other schools and colleges of the ZJU health care system, and the eight affiliated hospitals.[5] By pooling resources from these entities, the aim is to provide a world-class infrastructure with critical components of research support and quality control services. The two modules—research and clinical care—will be linked by the academic components of training for students in the MD, MS, and Ph.D. programs; translational and clinical research (including interdisciplinary components); and research-oriented clinical care.

ZJU leadership is concerned that the proposed ownership structure for the AMC, as described earlier, might not provide sufficient scope for collaboration between basic science researchers and clinical practitioners, as well as strong-enough mechanisms to support collaboration with computer scientists, big data experts, social scientists, and others needed to provide a fully interdisciplinary systems perspective on medical research. While the ownership structure will not change, ZJU is considering how to design key domains of the organizational structure, such as governance mechanisms, operational methods, and finances, to better meet their goals.

The purpose of this study is to provide advisory support for planning the organization of the ZJU AMC. In particular, RAND researchers were asked to identify and assess potential models of organization that could help the AMC achieve its goals.

---

[5]   The other schools and colleges that will participate in the AMC are envisaged to include the College of Computer Science and Technology, the College of Biomedical Engineering and Instrument Science, the School of Materials Science and Engineering, and the Department of Polymer Science and Engineering, among others.

CHAPTER TWO

Evaluation Criteria and Approach

In this chapter, we describe the evaluation criteria and approach we used to identify and ultimately rank the potential organizational models for ZJU to reasonably consider for its new AMC. In collaboration with the client, we carried out the following analysis:

1. We developed a logic model to identify and connect organizational domains and attributes with the specified outcomes of interest. As discussed in Chapter One, the outcomes of interest are innovation, quality, resource sustainability, and compliance.
2. We reviewed and identified organizational attributes that could help achieve the desired outcomes.
3. We reviewed and identified organizational domains that could help develop the desired organizational attributes.
4. We selected four U.S.-based AMCs as examples for developing case studies about the relationship between organizational domains, attributes, and outcomes.
5. We applied lessons from the case studies and our understanding of ZJU to develop a number of feasible models for an organizational structure. We then analyzed each model's strengths and weaknesses for achieving the desired attributes and ranked the models on likely performance.

Logic Model and Development of Organizational Domains

Our approach recognizes that organization structure is a key facilitator of outcomes through its rules and coordination mechanisms in all kinds of organizations.[1]

---

[1] For a discussion of organizational structure as a key facilitator of outcomes, see D. S. Pugh, *Organization Theory: Selected Readings*, Vol. 126, Harmondsworth, UK: Penguin, 1971; and John M. Bryson, *Strategic Planning for Public and Nonprofit Organizations: A Guide to Strengthening and Sustaining Organizational Achievement*, Hoboken, N.J.: John Wiley and Sons, 2011.

To understand which organizational components, particularly mechanisms for coordination and supervision, might best facilitate the outcomes of interest discussed in Chapter One, we use a logic model (see Figure 2.1).[2]

In our logic model, ownership, governance, identity, organizational policies, and organizational structure are inputs, which result in the production methods and attributes of the system to create outputs and, ultimately, outcomes. Organizational structure consists of rules and coordination mechanisms under which the organization's resources function in order to meet the system's goals.

Ownership. The owners of the organization are responsible not just to themselves but to a number of other stakeholders, such as user groups. In the case of the AMC, the user groups include students, employees, and patients. Owners respond to organizational stakeholders in a number of ways, which we describe next.

Governance. System owners select governance systems consisting of rules and coordination mechanisms that will guide the setting of policy. Governance systems are intended to address the interests of owners and other stakeholders.

Identity. The owners select an identity for the institution to meet stakeholder interests. The components of identity include the vision and mission of the organization, and the image and brand presented to stakeholders, both internal and external.[3]

Organizational policies. Organizational policies are a description of the outputs and outcomes to be achieved by the organization. Policies usually also specify the action plans required to achieve the results sought and the resources needed to fulfill the action plans.

Organizational structure. The organizational structure consists of rules and coordination mechanisms that will guide use of the system's resources. The mechanisms cause the organization to develop methods of providing goods and services, such as research methods and standards of clinical care.

Figure 2.1
Organizational Processes in a Logic Model

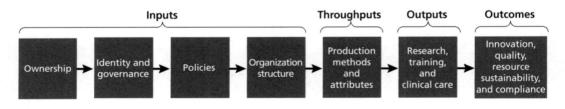

---

[2]   For a discussion of logic models, see Victoria Greenfield, Valerie L. Williams, and Elisa Eiseman, *Using Logic Models for Strategic Planning and Evaluation: Application to the National Center for Injury Prevention and Control*, Santa Monica, Calif.: RAND Corporation, TR-370-NCIPC, 2006. Logic models, when applied to operational control, focus on the rules under which the inputs of the organization interact.

[3]   See Appendix A for more information.

Attributes. Attributes refer to the characteristics of the production methods, such as the collaboration across disciplines in the production of research. The attributes are a part of organization culture, which consists of the "values, beliefs and assumptions . . . that define the way an organization operates."[4] They may be qualitative attributes, such as a commitment to organizational goals, or quantitative attributes, such as resource self-sufficiency. The production methods, based on resources and the attributes that guide them, lead to such outputs as clinical care, hopefully with the desired high-quality outcomes.

Within the above definition of organizational structure, the variations introduced by different levels of control of the AMC are of interest. A wide range of organizational structures exists. An AMC could be sponsored by (and therefore "owned" by) the sponsoring university, yet it could be organized as an independent entity for the purposes of its legal charter, with independent responsibility for appointing its board of trustees and for creating its own governance and operating entities. At the other extreme, the AMC could be a division of the SOM and entirely dependent on the SOM for fulfilling all AMC tasks, from devising governance systems to recruitment and finances. In between these extremes of dependence and autonomy, each organizational domain could take on characteristics of some dependence and some autonomy. The dependent components could be reliant on the SOM, one or more hospitals, or some combination of these.

Development of Organizational Attributes and Mapping Attributes to Outcomes

Existing research has identified the key attributes generated by an organization structure as commitment, loyalty, collaboration, communication, teamwork, and resource adequacy to promote professional growth.[5]

Applying these findings to the ZJU AMC, the RAND team developed a list of desired organizational attributes, as follows. The organization should:

1. Commit faculty, physicians, and affiliated entities to all AMC activities (clinical, research, teaching).
2. Leverage ZJU identity.
3. Promote functional integration, including
   a. integration of basic science, clinical, and translational research
   b. integration of clinical care and clinical research

---

[4] Jay B. Barney, "Organizational Culture: Can It Be a Source of Sustained Competitive Advantage?" *Academy of Management Review*, Vol. 11, No. 3, 1986, pp. 656–665.

[5] Chester I. Barnard, and Kenneth R. Andrews, *The Functions of the Executive*, Vol. 11, Cambridge, Mass.: Harvard University Press, 1968; Pugh, 1971.

      c.   integration of training and research

      d.   integration of clinical care and training.

5.   Promote interactions within ZJU, including within the AMC and affiliated entities.

6.   Promote collaborations between ZJU and external entities.

7.   Achieve financial stability, consisting of

      a.   adequate resources for training

      b.   adequate resources for research

      c.   adequate resources for clinical care

      d.   a cost-efficient pathway to establish the AMC.

Of course, not every attribute is equally important for each outcome. Some attributes, such as staff commitment, could be equally important for every outcome, while others, such as functional integration, might more directly affect innovation and quality while influencing resource sustainability only indirectly, and compliance perhaps not at all. However, in other attributes, such as financial stability, the influence on innovation could go either way, as the academic literature suggests.[6] In this case, we chose the more-traditional view in the literature of a positive influence. The attributes were mapped to outcomes as shown in Table 2.1.

In practice, measuring the organization's performance on attributes and outcomes can be challenging. Appropriate performance indicators need to be developed

Table 2.1
AMC Attributes Mapped to Outcomes

| Outcomes | Attributes | | | | | |
	Staff Commitment	ZJU Identity	Functional Integration	Interaction[a]	Collaboration[b]	Financial Stability
Innovation	X	X	X	X	X	X
Quality	X	X	X	X	X	X
Resource sustainability	X	X			X	X
Compliance[c]	X					X

[a] Interaction refers to internal interactions within ZJU, including within the AMC and affiliated entities.
[b] Collaboration refers to external collaborations.
[c] Compliance refers to compliance with local laws and regulations and capacity constraints.

---

[6]   Martin Hoegl, Michael Gibbert, and David Mazursky, "Financial Constraints in Innovation Projects: When Is Less More?" *Research Policy*, Vol. 37, No. 8, September 2008, pp. 1382–1391.

and, even then, measuring them may be difficult and contested. However, a consideration of this important aspect was beyond the scope of this report. We do, however, provide a discussion of approaches to monitoring performance in Chapter Seven.[7]

Case Study Selection

After a review of several highly ranked SOMs in the United States, RAND researchers identified four for more detailed study. See Appendix B for the selection procedure. The selected SOMs are organized as AMCs and are global leaders in academic medicine. They were selected with a careful eye toward identifying AMCs with varying organizational models for integrating research, clinical practice, and teaching. Before final selection of the cases, we talked to contacts at each site to understand how their AMCs were organized, to ensure that there was enough variation in organizational domains within the group to derive useful conclusions. We also reviewed the short list with ZJU.

In the case studies, we focused on understanding the organizational structure of the AMCs and how the mechanisms influenced the development of desired organizational attributes.

The AMCs selected for the case studies were

- Harvard Medical School (HMS) and its affiliates
- Stanford Medicine
- University of California, Los Angeles (UCLA) Health
- University of Washington (UW) Medicine.

We reviewed publicly available evidence and held discussions with key informants from these AMCs to (1) determine how their systems might be applied to ZJU and where the entire model may not apply to ZJU and (2) to identify specific factors that might be appropriate for adoption. Specifically, we sought to understand the ownership and identity, governance and operations, and finances for each system. We also dedicated time during discussions to elicit discussants' views of strengths and gaps in their own organization and governance systems.

Beyond simply understanding the features of the various systems, we tried to understand how adoption of a specific organizational structure would serve the goals of ZJU. The literature on AMC governance highlights the importance of context and history in the design of strong governance systems.[8] The research shows that having

---

[7] For a discussion of performance indicators, see Roberto Mosse and Leigh Ellen Sontheimer, *Performance Monitoring Indicators Handbook (English)*, Washington, D.C.: World Bank, Technical Paper No. 334, 1996.

[8] Gregory R. Wegner, "Academic Health Center Governance and the Responsibilities of University Boards and Chief Executives (Report of a Symposium)," Washington, D.C.: Association of Governing Boards of Universities

designated leadership in each area (e.g., medical care, education, research) that is also aligned with the overall vision of the AMC can help reduce conflict while enhancing sound decisionmaking. [9] The research also suggests that decisionmaking is improved with the establishment of governing and operating entities with specific expertise, including boards with specific knowledge about local contextual factors.[10]

In addition, real-world experience with implementation informs the need to ensure that the model is flexible and agile in order to respond to new insights; able to mobilize partners throughout the organization where needed; and able to forge and hold together coalitions—i.e., get people to agree to something and then stick with it long enough to make it happen.[11] Therefore, where possible, we also sought to understand how these models came into existence.

Applying the Lessons and Recommending Organizational Models

The case studies provided lessons on the differences and similarities between the four models studied. We used these findings to derive more general conclusions regarding the importance of each organizational domain considered and the relationship between organizational domains and the achievement of attributes.

The next step in our approach was to develop and compare models differentiated by organizational structures that could influence the attributes in a desirable direction. This led to a ranking of the models in order of likely performance of the attributes. Based on these rankings, we recommended a preferred model. We also suggested a second choice as an interim alternative with the ultimate goal of implementing the preferred model.

---

and Colleges, Occasional Paper 50, 2003.

[9]   Adrianna Kezar and Peter D. Eckel, "Meeting Today's Governance Challenges: A Synthesis of the Literature and Examination of a Future Agenda for Scholarship," *Journal of Higher Education*, Vol. 75, No. 4, July–August 2004, pp. 371–399.

[10]   M. J. Kurtz and A. Schrank, "Growth and Governance: Models, Measures, and Mechanisms," *Journal of Politics*, Vol. 69, No. 2, May 2007, pp. 538–554.

[11]   See, for example, Richard E. Matland, "Synthesizing the Implementation Literature: The Ambiguity-Conflict Model of Policy Implementation," *Journal of Public Administration Research and Theory*, Vol. 5, No. 2, April 1995, pp. 145–174; C. Blakely, J. Meyer, R. Gottschalk, N. Schmidt, W. Davidson, D. Roitman, and J. Emshoff, "The Fidelity-Adaptation Debate: Implications for the Implementation of Public Sector Social Programs," *American Journal of Community Psychology*, Vol. 15, No. 3, 1987; Susan J. Bodilly, Thomas K. Glennan, Jr., Kerri A. Kerr, and Jolene Galegher, "Introduction: Framing the Problem," in Thomas K. Glennan, Jr., Susan J. Bodilly, Jolene Galegher, and Kerri A. Kerr, *Expanding the Reach of Education Reforms: Perspectives from Leaders in the Scale-Up of Educational Interventions*, Santa Monica, Calif.: RAND Corporation, MG-248-FF, 2004, pp. 1–40.

CHAPTER THREE

Case Studies

Overview

As noted in Chapter Two, the AMCs that we selected for further study incorporate the SOM, other professional health care schools, and one or more hospitals. Either in practice or intent, the AMCs we studied encompass all the health care activities of a university and its clinical care affiliates, with a high level of integration between them. Through such integrated work, AMCs provide vital clinical care, conduct cutting-edge research, and educate the nation's future health care workforce.

In this chapter, we describe four AMCs that are among the global leaders in academic medicine in the United States:[1]

- HMS and its affiliates
- Stanford Medicine
- UCLA Health
- UW Medicine.

For each AMC, we provide a brief summary that describes the ownership and identity, governance and operations, and finances for each system.

HMS and its Affiliates

HMS is part of Harvard University in Cambridge, Massachusetts, and has 17 affiliated hospitals and institutes.[2] Although there are other AMCs in the United States that have a similar general structure, the specifics of the arrangements between HMS and affiliated hospitals are relatively unusual. This is in large part due to HMS's long

---

[1]   The medical schools of Harvard University, Stanford University, UCLA, and UW were ranked No. 1, No. 4, No. 7 and No. 24, respectively, in the world in 2018 by QS Top Universities (see QS, "QS World University Rankings: Medicine," webpage, undated). UW is the biggest recipient of research funding among public universities.

[2]   Harvard Medical School, "HMS Affiliates," webpage, undated.

history, some of which predates the formation of the United States itself, and also due in part to its global preeminence. One of our interviewees noted that "nobody would purposefully design a system like this from scratch." Nevertheless, given its stature as the world's leading AMC, there could be important insights to be gleaned from examining this model.

Ownership and Identity

HMS and each of its affiliated hospitals are separate financial and legal entities. Moreover, each hospital is a principal investigating unit that subcontracts with the other institutions within the system for collaborations and has its own IRB for human subjects research.

Governance and Operations

There is a high degree of competition among the HMS-affiliated hospitals, as many are full-service general hospitals and provide duplicative services. At the same time, HMS is charged with fostering community among faculty. The vast majority of HMS faculty (totaling approximately 10,000) are employed by one of the affiliated hospitals, not by HMS. A small minority of HMS faculty, largely nonclinical researchers (usually Ph.D.s without MDs), are employed only by HMS and do not have additional appointments or employment at one of the affiliated hospitals.

This system works because hospital staff want to be faculty within the HMS system. Despite HMS being in a financially weak position compared with any of the affiliated hospitals,[3] HMS affiliation provides access to the Harvard name, thus enabling the affiliate to be part of one of the preeminent universities in the world. This makes it a magnet for the highest-quality medical graduates, residents, and faculty. The result is a synergistic relationship between hospital and medical school in which the hospitals need HMS because it provides access to the Harvard brand and confers status (professorship) to their employees. In turn, HMS needs the hospitals for access to teaching and research faculty and, sometimes, capital. This synergy occurs despite organizational and financial tensions between the institutions.

HMS's power in the relationship centers on its ability to confer HMS faculty appointments and promotions which, as noted earlier, bring considerable prestige and, with it, access to "the best" faculty and students. By requirement of the Harvard affiliation agreement, every doctor at the affiliated hospitals must be a faculty member of HMS. Faculty are employed on the clinical, research, or teaching tracks, or some combination thereof. Faculty appointments require approval of the medical school's executive committee (EC). Each HMS clinical department (e.g., medicine, surgery) has an EC that reports to the HMS Dean. The EC for each department consists of the chairs

---

[3]   Luke W. Vrotsos, "White Coats Face Red Balance Sheets at Harvard Medical School," *Harvard Crimson*, May 23, 2018.

of those departments at each hospital (e.g., the EC for Medicine includes the Chairs of Medicine at the Brigham and Women's Hospital, Massachusetts General Hospital, Mount Auburn Hospital).

Lower-level faculty appointments usually involve only a cursory review by the EC. However, promotions to the associate or full professor level at any of the affiliate hospitals require more extensive reviews by an EC. High-profile appointments may require even more review. For instance, a search for a new head of a cardiology department at one of the hospitals requires a separate search committee comprised of other associate and full professors, mostly from the hiring hospital but also from other hospitals. This confers ongoing brand consistency, because nonprofessors cannot promote professors.

HMS faculty who are employed at the hospitals and paid virtually nothing by HMS perform nearly 70 percent of the teaching in the first two years of medical school and all teaching in the last two years of HMS. Instead, funding to compensate those faculty comes from the clinical departments at their own hospitals. These investments are made in order to maintain access to the HMS brand name and, therefore, access to high caliber residents and faculty. Other AMCs may do substantial recruitment from the outside, but because of the pull of Harvard, many people who train at Harvard-affiliated hospitals want to remain within the system.

Finances

It is important to note that HMS does not have access to clinical income. Its only revenue is from tuition, endowments, or grants won by the small minority of HMS-only faculty members. The research budgets of the affiliated hospitals are much bigger than HMS's research budget. HMS receives approximately $250 million to $350 million in National Institutes of Health (NIH) annual funding. In comparison, Partners Healthcare (a health system consisting of HMS affiliates Brigham and Women's Hospital, Massachusetts General Hospital, Massachusetts Eye and Ear, McLean Hospital, and Spaulding Rehabilitation Hospital) receives about $800 million.

Because of this imbalance in funding levels, HMS may call on some hospital resources. Occasionally, the hospitals will transfer funds to HMS to cover some costs, but these transfers are not done regularly or systematically. In addition, these transfers are usually too small, irregular, and insufficient for the medical school to embark on large-scale projects in an autonomous way.

However, HMS is able to report the collective funding of all the hospitals when reporting NIH funding figures, which affects academic rankings. Moreover, while hospitals have their own labs, there are no major distinctions between the types of research being done at the affiliated hospitals and work being done at HMS itself (although more clinically oriented work is likely to be done by hospital-based faculty in hospital laboratories). In addition, there are large collaborative grants that include both HMS and hospitals, including some very large grant-funded initiatives like the Dana Farber Cancer Institute and the Translational Research Center.

In contrast, the hospitals are generally well funded and have multiple mechanisms for keeping the institution running, including large amounts of grant funding, receptive bond markets (largely for funding infrastructure improvements), and philanthropy (because big donors are generally those who are satisfied with the clinical care they received). These sources are in addition to the hospitals' main sources of revenue, which are for clinical care and professional consultations and come from various insurance programs.

Stanford Medicine

At Stanford University, the SOM and its affiliated hospitals, including Stanford Hospital, make up the AMC.

Ownership and Identity

The SOM is owned by the university, governed by the university's rules, and employs its own faculty. The hospital is owned by the university, but it is not governed by the university's rules. Instead, it has its own charter, board of trustees, and legal structure. Its employees are hospital employees, not university employees.

The independent structure offers the hospital the advantages of having its own human resources structure and its own financial and operating structure, which simplifies and speeds up decisionmaking. For example, Stanford Hospital has recently been buying smaller hospitals to gain market share. For this, it does not need to obtain university approval. This can be beneficial because, in many instances, universities have slow, bureaucratic decisionmaking processes, whereas hospitals must make many rapid-turnaround decisions. Separate legal and financial structures facilitate more timely decisionmaking.

Similarly, the SOM is able to make strategic decisions that take into account its own particular contextual factors. For instance, one issue used to be getting younger faculty to participate in hospital activities, such as clinical and teaching duties. This was difficult in the past given that most younger faculty focused on research and teaching to gain tenure, leaving the hospital with insufficient human capital. This has improved in recent years. Now, most Stanford SOM faculty are hired in nontenure track positions under different lines. However, they may receive other privileges—for example, the ability to buy a home on campus (Stanford University and Stanford Hospital are located in extremely high-cost areas).

Governance and Operations

The staff of the affiliated hospitals may seek an affiliation with the SOM, but they are not required to be affiliated with the SOM or be hired with the consultation of the SOM. Therefore, the arrangements under which the Stanford AMC runs differ from

Harvard in terms of the role it plays in hiring staff at the hospitals. As with HMS, the independent legal structure exists because hospitals are, unlike universities, revenue-generating operations that are organized as nonprofits and earn revenue for providing clinical care from patients, insurance companies, and the government.

This relatively decentralized decisionmaking process carries over into individual hospital departments. Within Stanford Hospital, the organizational structure is intended to enable quasi-autonomous departments—for example, the department of neurology and the department of surgery, each with its own management structure in charge of departmental finances, space, and recruitment. The hospital "leases" out its space to departments based on budgets.

There are numerous collaborations between the hospital and the SOM, as well as with other nonmedical departments (e.g., engineering). This is encouraged by Stanford University, its SOM, and the hospitals and is believed to be very successful to date. Students also mediate such collaborations. For example, the course "Anatomy for Bio-engineers" frames an engineering problem around anatomical issues. Students, who include engineers and SOM students, might be given a cadaveric knee joint and a prosthetic knee joint and asked to analyze the differences and why these exist. The hospital also supports the devices department within SOM. The Bio-X initiative, which focuses on interdisciplinary work through research seminars, also provides such shared infrastructure as 3-D printing.

Finances

The SOM receives revenue through tuition and research grants. Most basic science research labs are located in the SOM. If a hospital physician wishes to undertake research using the facilities of the SOM, a fee is typically paid by the hospital's department to the lab, usually captured as part of the overhead charge in a grant application. Those who conduct both clinical work in the hospital and research at the SOM will typically negotiate the share of time spent at each facility, with salaries calculated accordingly.

In addition, each hospital department pays a share of its revenue to the SOM (a so-called Dean's Tax) to support the long-term development of the SOM. At Stanford, each hospital department negotiates its revenue share with the SOM.[4] The revenue share may be a percentage or may be based on a flat fee with some variation based on revenue. Typically, this results in a revenue share of 3 percent to 7 percent.

The hospital—not the SOM—funds residency training (known as graduate medical education). At the backend, the hospital may receive federal funding to help support this. In the past, federal funding, such as the U.S. Department of Veterans Affairs funding and Center for Medicare and Medicaid Services funding, provided

---

[4]   In other AMCs, this may be negotiated between the SOM and the hospital as a whole.

most of the funds for resident training, but the share has been declining and the difference is being borne by the hospital's own funds.

Salaries in the SOM are generally lower than hospital salaries. When SOM faculty provide services to the hospital, the hospital compensates the SOM based on a Medicare rate known as the Relative Value Unit. It is the same rate used for compensating physicians employed by the hospital—capturing procedures, complexity, and risk coverage. A typical physician's salary will include base pay, incentives for good outcomes and quantity of work done, and bonuses based on the hospital's overall performance, among other factors.

UCLA Health

At UCLA, four hospitals and an SOM comprise its AMC.

Ownership and Identity

UCLA owns four hospitals within the AMC. Of these, Ronald Reagan Medical Center (RRMC) is the largest, with an annual revenue of $5 billion. In the past and up to the present time, the hospital and its SOM (the David Geffen School of Medicine [DGSOM]) have been independent financial entities, with their own staff and infrastructure. As with Stanford's AMC, affiliated hospitals' staff may seek an affiliation with the SOM, but they are not required to be affiliated with the SOM or to be hired with the consultation of the SOM.

Governance and Operations

There is a general goal of greater collaboration between the DGSOM and RRMC (which are physically proximate to each other). This begins with the leadership of both institutions, who confer regularly to define areas of collaboration. At present, education and all research, excluding clinical research, are managed by DGSOM or an affiliated university entity, such as the School of Nursing, while the management of clinical care resides in the RRMC. The long-term strategic plan calls for integration of all these functions. Furthermore, there are forums and mechanisms for interaction—for example, a new structure known as the President's Council, where all the clinical chairs provide feedback on how to work together; this is captured in documents and shared. There is no fixed time line to complete integration; this is envisaged to be a years-long journey, with an initial focus on functional integration and with financial integration at the end.

Similar to Stanford, the medical students are fully administered by the SOM, take all their coursework at the SOM, and have rotations in the hospital. Unlike Stanford, the residency program is administered and funded by the SOM, in collaboration with the respective clinical departments. There is currently no natural incentive for

SOM faculty to be involved in the hospital. Some only see a handful of patients each year and spend most of their time on teaching or, more commonly, research. There are also concerns about the link between clinical research and care. In 2013, UCLA appointed a chief medical officer (CMO) for clinical research, with the goal of serving as the bridge between clinical research and patient care.

Clinical research is usually initiated within RRMC and may involve faculty from DGSOM. Financial incentives drive physicians to prioritize clinical care over research because their salaries are based on metrics of clinical care. This contributes to low integration between the research activities of physicians of RRMC and the faculty of DGSOM. Still, the perception conveyed by interviewees is that increased integration is beginning to happen. However, it often exists only at the departmental level and the degree to which this occurs varies across departments. One common model for some departments is that the practitioner needs to meet a threshold in clinical earnings and can allocate time as desired thereafter (e.g., to teaching, research, or administrative work).

One way to increase attention to nonclinical research is to gear recruitment toward physician-researchers. In practice, however, recruitment practices vary significantly and are dependent on the needs of various departments. Developing multidisciplinary work, incorporating innovative technologies, and initiating translational research is a challenge in most institutions. An investment fund has been established under the leadership of a senior director of research and innovation for RRMC and the SOM. This individual provides an organizational bridge that supports transformational initiatives focused on research innovation and commercialization. The physical proximity of RRMC to the SOM and its location within the UCLA campus comes with advantages and can foster participation and collaboration between basic science and clinical research.

Finances

The RRMC provides financial support to SOM of several million U.S. dollars on an annual basis. As with Stanford, the SOM also captures a Dean's Tax, which is a share of RRMC revenue determined mutually between the SOM and individual clinical departments within the RRMC. This is essentially a tax on physicians' revenue, and it ranges from 10 percent to 36 percent of a department's clinical earnings. It mostly derives from professional fees and does not include insurance reimbursements or grants.

There is no clear or consistent gap in salary between SOM faculty and hospital physicians. Physicians typically earn more, but the salary does vary widely by different specializations and departments. A 10-to-30-percent range is probably typical.

UW Medicine

At UW, the AMC consists of four hospitals, an SOM, neighborhood clinics, an airlift unit, and a clinical practice group.

Ownership and Identity
The university owns all the components of the UW AMC. The clinical care components are branded with the UW identity.

Governance and Operations
The leaders of the major clinical programs at the UW Health System report to the CMO of the UW Health System. The teaching and basic science departments are overseen by their department chairs, who in turn report to the Dean of the SOM through the vice deans of research and education. The CMO supports the integration of hospital and university policies through a committee that includes the vice deans and heads of clinical programs.

All staff are recruited and employed by the SOM, and the hospitals pay a fee to the SOM for staff time spent doing clinical activities.

The SOM is organized into departments, including several clinical departments (e.g., medicine and surgery), basic science, and research centers or institutions. Most SOM staff who are attached to clinical departments also work clinically within those departments (typically 65 percent to 70 percent of their time), with the remainder of the time allocated to teaching, research, or some combination thereof, as agreed upon with the corresponding department chair. Nonclinical SOM staff do not typically work clinically, but they may perform basic science research within the SOM.

Finances
Under this model, the hospitals generate revenue, mainly from clinical care. They pay a Dean's Tax (about 11 percent) to support the overall enterprise managed by the SOM. Revenues for the SOM include tuition and fees from students, physicians' professional consultation fees (currently about $400 million a year), plus a share of the hospital's revenue (currently about $235 million a year). In addition, the Relative Value Unit concept at Stanford—to compensate SOM faculty who provide clinical care—also applies to UW faculty. Because all staff are employees of the SOM, this arrangement covers all staff. Furthermore, all research grants, including clinical research grants, come through the SOM.

As a general indicator of success, UW is the recipient of the highest amount of NIH funds among public universities in the United States (about $700 million a year). It also obtains research funding from the private sector, while providing a significant amount of free or subsidized care as a public institution.

Differences and Similarities Among the AMCs

There are some important differences and similarities among the four AMCs, but we found no simple differentiator among them. Table 3.1 maps the entities that are the main drivers of different operational activities.

As discussed earlier, ownership and identity, governance and operations, and finances are believed to be key facilitators of performance. We now discuss how these domains compare across the case studies and what we may learn about their influence on desired system attributes.

Ownership and Identity

The Harvard system, which has many independent affiliated hospitals, each with its own ownership structure, differs in ownership when compared with the other three AMCs, all of which own their hospitals. This, in turn, has led to a greater sense of focused identity around the university's brand in the other three AMCs relative to Harvard. This appears to generate greater commitment among stakeholders toward common shared goals of the system in these three systems. Therefore, the findings in regard to ownership and identity from the case studies reinforce their importance in

Table 3.1
Entities Mapped to Operations in the Case Studies

Operational Activities	AMC			
	Harvard	Stanford	UCLA	UW
Clinical research	Hospital (driven)	Hospital	Hospital	AMC
Basic science, interdisciplinary, and translational research	SOM	SOM	SOM	AMC
Training MDs	• Pre-clinical: hospital • Clinical: hospital	• Pre-clinical: SOM • Clinical: hospital	• Pre-clinical: SOM • Clinical: hospital	AMC
Training MSs and Ph.D.s	SOM	SOM	SOM	SOM
Clinical care	• Recruitment and evaluation: SOM and hospital • Allocation and monitoring: hospital	Hospital	Hospital	• Recruitment, allocation and evaluation: AMC • Monitoring: hospital
External collaboration	No institutional driver. In some cases, external grant funding entities (e.g., NIH) seek to encourage collaboration and have funding mechanisms with that explicit goal.			

facilitating the achievement of two desired attributes, stakeholder commitment and leveraging the university's identity.

Governance and Operations

A common factor among the cases studied is shared governance. This seems to reflect a common understanding that sharing governance enables expertise from diverse sources to be pooled—i.e., it promotes functional integration. Shared governance also creates positive incentives for stakeholder commitment to the system.

The extent of such shared governance varies in formality—for example, at UW, there is a CMO who chairs a committee of deans and clinical department heads and is formally empowered with a mandate to integrate governance; whereas at UCLA, governance is shared informally through the President's Council.

Stanford has made several efforts to move from a sharing of governance responsibilities to greater integration. The Bio-X initiative is its most notable initiative in this respect. Integrating governance at Stanford is arguably easier than at UCLA, because UCLA offers a much wider range of specializations and more-comprehensive care than Stanford does.

The importance of shared governance as a common factor across all four AMCs stands in contrast to the high variation observed regarding operational control between the four case studies. In terms of recruitment and other operational matters, UW has awarded significant control to the SOM. For example, all physicians are university employees, and decisions on the allocation of their time are made jointly by the SOM and hospital. Harvard also holds significant control over physician recruitment to its SOM, with all appointments at the affiliated hospitals requiring the SOM's approval, in return for which the appointee obtains faculty status at the university. However, the physicians are employees of their hospitals. For other operational matters, such as infrastructure decisions and resource-raising, the hospitals and the SOM act independently of each other. Operational control at the Stanford and UCLA AMCs is even more decentralized than at Harvard. Aside from independent decisionmaking regarding infrastructure and other operational matters, hospitals recruit physicians independently of the SOM.

The case studies show that, with regard to operational control, all four AMCs share some responsibilities between entities. A shared system requires greater interaction and collaboration among the entities of the system and with external entities, thus addressing key desired attributes of the system. However, aligning a shared system across both governance and operations, with a leading role for the SOM (as at UW), appears to create the most suitable incentives for functional integration and collaboration.

Finances

The Harvard system provides its SOM the least financial stability, with its revenue coming from student fees, university grants, and external grants. The most-lucrative components of the system (i.e., the insurance payments and professional fees) are retained by the hospitals. The hospitals compete with each other and with the SOM for clinical research funding, and they have historically been more successful at receiving such funding than the SOM. However, by tradition, the hospitals offer clinical training to the SOM's MD students. Furthermore, the large number, high quality, and diversity of affiliated hospitals are an advantage for the SOM, as this enables the SOM to participate in its research grants and give its students and residents access to a large number of mentors and diverse fields of research and care.

The UCLA and Stanford AMCs are similar in their financial dependence on the hospitals. Although owned by the universities, their hospitals are operated as independent trusts and make their own decisions with regard to resource-raising and spending. The SOMs in both AMCs are able to institutionalize some financial transfers from the hospitals to themselves through the Dean's Tax, and they retain a large faculty base that participates in clinical care and research and thus earns revenue for the SOM.

Both Stanford and UCLA view the transfer of resources from the hospital to the SOM as necessary to support the long-term development of the SOM and to offset current account deficits. Both face the challenge of financially weaker SOMs seeking to integrate with financially strong hospitals.

UW is the most stable financial system due to the access of the SOM to large, guaranteed revenue sources. The perception internally at UW is that this structure, modeled on another prestigious institution (the University of California, San Francisco), has played a key role in ensuring attention to all components of the system, as well as ensuring that these components are coordinated and allow for a balanced approach toward teaching, research, and patient care.

The differences in financial stability show up in the resources available for different activities. The large financial capacity of the hospitals supports a high level of resources for clinical research in the Harvard system, but activities that are limited to the university can be resource-constrained. This is most noticeable in the training functions of the university, with the HMS relying on the largesse of the hospitals for accomplishing much of its training functions. UW appears to be the best positioned in this respect.

There is an important lesson here for ZJU. The financial instability that affects HMS may be affordable because of the reputation and wealth of Harvard University as a whole. For ZJU's AMC, such a model is less likely to be successful. Therefore, it is important for ZJU to find an organization structure that offers financial stability.

However, this can be a challenge because of the differences in scale and staff status between the hospital and the SOM—a situation that is common globally, including at ZJU. The hospitals are typically large entities with an assured source of revenue from clinical care that covers costs, while the SOMs typically have much smaller operating budgets and run a deficit. Physicians at a hospital typically earn more than faculty at an SOM and have an implicit assurance of long-term contracts. For faculty, long-term contracts are given only to the small fraction of staff with tenure. As in the case of Stanford Medicine, even this is changing, as most SOM faculty are now hired to non-tenure track positions in exchange for other, potentially equally desirable benefits (e.g., access to affordable housing in a high-cost area).

The rapid rise in international rankings of two more-recently formed schools—UCLA and UW medical schools were both founded in 1945, compared with Stanford (established in 1858) and Harvard (established in 1782)—shows that it is possible for schools to quickly rise in quality. Both UCLA and UW benefited from offering comprehensive health science studies, covering all the major disciplines; and from the presence, from their early days, of physically proximate and organizationally linked comprehensive clinical care facilities. Further, as public universities designated as flagship institutions in their regions, they received strong government support. Perhaps as important, in both cases, support from private donors joined with government support to play an important role. Major donors included the Hollywood businessman David Geffen (in the case of UCLA) and the Bill and Melinda Gates Foundation (in the case of UW).

The case studies show that a shared approach to financial management can lead to financial fragility and uncertainty unless the SOM is empowered to play a guiding role (as at UW). To achieve financial stability, which we identified as a desirable attribute, an important role for the SOM seems to be required.

Table 3.2 summarizes the differences between the case studies in their organizational domains.

Table 3.2
Organizational Structures of the Case Studies

Case Studies	Ownership	Identity	Governance	Operational Control	Finances
UW	University	University	Shared	Shared	University
Stanford University and UCLA	University	University	Shared	Shared	Shared
Harvard University	Divided	Shared	Shared	Shared	Shared

CHAPTER FOUR

Organizational Model Development

In Chapter Three, we discussed four cases of leading AMCs in the United States and derived lessons about how organizational domains influenced performance. In this chapter, we apply our findings to discuss how the key domains of AMC organizational structure (ownership and identity, governance and operations, and finances) influence the desired attributes of organizational processes in the context of the ZJU AMC.

Ownership and Identity

Although none of the goals ZJU articulated fall under the domain of ownership, it is an important contextual factor to consider, particularly in situations in which ownership of certain activities may need to change to establish certain models.

An important role of ownership is specifying the AMC's identity, which includes specifying the vision, mission, and image to external stakeholders. In three of the AMCs we studied—UW, UCLA, and Stanford—the leading entity (e.g., SOM, AMC) imparts its identity on the subsidiary entities within the organization.

In the case of Harvard, despite divided ownership, a common identity is sought (though this faces challenges) as it appears to hold great value for all entities. The entities that are not owned by Harvard (e.g., affiliated hospitals) have been willing to negotiate on such factors as control over faculty appointments and promotions in order to share in that identity. HMS also gains from sharing its identity with the hospitals in fundraising and in enabling its students to access a wide range of clinical care environments.

In the case of UW, the entire AMC enterprise shares a single identity, which may help align priorities across potentially disparate subsidiary entities (e.g., the hospital and the SOM). For Stanford and UCLA, despite their operational independence, the hospitals have been willing to relinquish some control over revenue (through the Dean's Tax and other transfers) in return for sharing the university's identity. As discussed earlier, a common identity appears to generate commitment among stakeholders toward the goals of the system, potentially even when sacrifices are involved.

These cases suggest that successfully building a distinct common identity around the name of ZJU (to which all its entities can commit to) could help the ZJU AMC in various ways, particularly in stakeholder commitment. Building a common identity emerges as a goal of each of the institutions in the case studies, even when ownership is divided. This shows the importance of a common identity. The case studies also show that it is possible to strive for a common identity even when ownership is divided.

For ZJU, the desired attributes that could result from a common identity include the opportunity to

- obtain the commitment of faculty, physicians, and affiliated entities to all activities of the AMC
- leverage the ZJU identity.

Governance and Operations

From the case studies, we learned that all four AMCs adopted a shared governance system that is broadly similar across the cases, with some variation in the degree of formality in the structures. By contrast, there is greater variation in the sharing of operational control. While all four AMCs share some responsibilities between entities, the UW system, which is the most formal and which assigns a leading role for the SOM, appears to create the most suitable incentives for functional integration and collaboration.

The cases suggest that building a shared governance and operations system at ZJU, with a guiding role for the SOM, creates the opportunity to influence the following attributes:

- functional integration
- interactions within ZJU, including within the AMC and affiliated entities
- collaborations between ZJU and external entities.

Finances

As the case studies showed, the stability and sustainability of financial resources are not assured. This is due to the volatility of certain kinds of revenue and the costs of running certain operations. Revenue from clinical care (patient care) and student training are relatively stable sources of revenue, while research grants are less stable. Clinical care is a more sustainable activity, in that revenues cover costs once the system stabilizes. Student training rarely generates sufficient income through tuition to cover costs, but it brings brand value, a potential pipeline for recruitment, and other long-term benefits, both to the institution and society. Research is usually sustainable over the long term, in the sense that researchers are usually expected to raise enough revenue to cover their costs, but research is less likely to be sustainable when the institution is new because researchers will be also be new to the institution and need time to establish or re-establish themselves.

Achieving financial stability in the cases studied emerged as a challenge even at the most prestigious institutions. The cases suggest that the organizational model that is likely to work best for ZJU is one that requires all revenue to be pooled and spending to be allocated from the pool regardless of the source of funds. Furthermore, allocating the lead role to the SOM appears to be important. If these conditions are met, the AMC system could derive the following advantages:

- financial stability
- adequate resources for training
- adequate resources for research
- adequate resources for clinical care
- a cost-efficient pathway to establish the AMC.

Deriving Organizational Structure Models

Although feasible models of organization could lie anywhere on the spectrum of these identified organizational domains, we identified four specific models with variations in these domains and that warrant further analysis that could reasonably be considered by ZJU for governance of the new AMC.

To derive these models, we first explored all the different possible organizational structures suggested by the case studies. As Table 3.2 shows, there is considerable variation in organizational structure, thus enabling a rich comparison of the effects of organizational structure on attribute development and outcomes.

Missing from our case studies, however, is a common and successful AMC structure, both in the United States and elsewhere: the hospital-owned and -operated AMC. This is unlike the four AMCs studied, all of which are either university-owned or in which ownership is divided between the university and the hospital.

To address this gap, we reviewed material provided to us by ZJU on Charite-Berlin University's AMC, which is a hospital-owned and operated AMC. We have included its organizational structure as one of the four models under consideration.

In addition, we considered and deleted those organizational models that were not consistent with ZJU's constraints. The two constraints are that ownership of the AMC's components are divided between the SOM and the hospital, and that the identity of the AMC must be built around the identity of ZJU. See Appendix A for the analysis.

The following models emerged from the above filters:

1. **An autonomous model (or AMC-led model)**, in which ownership is divided between the university and the hospital and governance is shared between the university and the hospital. The AMC adopts the identity of the university and operates autonomously.
2. **A hospital-led model**, in which ownership is divided between the university and the hospital and governance is shared between the university and the hospital. The AMC adopts the identity of the hospital and is operated by the hospital.
3. **A shared model**, in which ownership is divided between the university and the hospital and governance is shared between the university and the hospital. The AMC adopts the identity of the university and is operated jointly by the hospital and the university. The AMC's training functions are owned by the university and operated by the SOM. The AMC's clinical care functions are owned and operated by an affiliated hospital. Research ownership and operation vary by type. Basic science, translational, and interdisciplinary research are owned and operated by the university and operated by the SOM, and clinical research is owned and operated by the hospital. The university imparts its identity to the AMC, including the academic activities, clinical care, and clinical research functions.
4. **A university-led model**, in which ownership is divided between the university and the hospital and governance is shared between the university and the hospital. The AMC adopts the identity of the university and is operated by the university.

We note that there may be further variations within the above models. For example, in the shared model, the hospital might adopt some parts of the university's identity, such as its brand name, when applying for research funds. However, the hospital might retain its own identity for other purposes, such as clinical care. In the university-led model, the hospital and SOM might identify themselves as independent of each other and compete in some respects, typically for research funding and recruitment; or the university might assign the guiding role to the SOM for shaping brand identity.

In Chapter Five, we describe these four system types based on how they perform in each of the key domains (ownership and identity, governance and operations, and finances) and through an assessment of strengths and weaknesses describe each model's contribution to achieving desired attributes and outcomes. From this analysis, we identify the models that, based on the evidence at hand, are best able to address the challenges ZJU faces while capitalizing on existing strengths.

CHAPTER FIVE

Assessment of Organizational System Models and Recommendations

Overview

In all four models of organizational structure discussed in Chapter Four, ownership is divided between the university and the hospital, while governance is shared between the university and the hospital. The differences between the models lie in identity and operational control.

The four models differ in the following respects:

1. In the **AMC-led model**, the AMC adopts the identity of the university and operates autonomously
2. In the **hospital-led model**, the AMC adopts the identity of the hospital and is operated by the hospital.
3. In the **shared model**, the AMC adopts the identity of the university and is operated jointly by the hospital and the university.
4. In the **university-led model**, the AMC adopts the identity of the university and is operated by the university.

In this chapter, we compare the models on key organizational domains. We also discuss how each system might be established or initiated, and its strengths and weaknesses with regard to achieving the desired attributes of the AMC.

AMC-Led Model

Under this system, the AMC has its own independent operational status. The UW system is most similar to this AMC-led model. However, the UW system model also has similarities to the university-led system discussed later in this chapter.

Ownership and Identity

Under such a system, the AMC is a unit owned partly by the university (research and training) and partly by a hospital (clinical care functions). It is operationally independent of the existing SOM and hospitals. The AMC adopts the identity of the university.

Governance and Operations

A university-appointed board of trustees provides governance. The board of trustees includes representation from the SOM and the hospitals. The AMC board of trustees selects the executive leadership of the AMC, including the chief executive officer (CEO). The AMC staff are university employees.

As a stand-alone unit, the AMC contains all the essential functions of an academic medical system (i.e., training, research, and care). These functions are divided among the AMC's suborganizational divisions, which consist of an SOM division (AMC-SOM), a hospital division (AMC-H), and a research division (AMC-R).

The AMC-SOM manages education and training as its core activity, and the AMC-H manages clinical care as its core activity. Research is managed as an independent activity of the AMC, under the AMC-R. The AMC-SOM, AMC-H, and AMC-R could be further operationally decentralized in order to enable autonomous functioning and meet statutory requirements. For example, each division could have its own management structure in charge of recruitment, operations, space, and finances. Furthermore, the AMC-SOM and AMC-H could choose to enter into contractual relations with the SOM and affiliated hospitals for linkages in recruitment, training, certification, research, and care.[1]

Finances

The AMC-H generates revenues primarily from clinical care, which is largely funded by the fees charged for clinical services. The AMC-SOM's core activity is training, which is funded by student fees and AMC support. The AMC manages all research functions under the AMC-R under the supervision of the Dean of Research and funded by research grants.

The AMC-H, AMC-SOM, and AMC-R pool net revenues, after meeting clinical care costs of the AMC-H, costs of training of the AMC-SOM, and costs of research for the AMC-R. The surplus, if any, is used to foster collaborations, innovation, and other desired growth initiatives.

Establishment

Establishment of an AMC-led system could be time-consuming and costly relative to the other AMCs. This is because the AMC would assume the sole responsibilities

---

[1]   In principle, the AMC-SOM and AMC-H may enter into contractual relations with any entity, domestically and internationally.

for resource-raising, hiring, and other factors that are shared in the other models. In addition, there might be capacity constraints at the AMC, which could limit what it is able to do.

Strengths and Weaknesses of the Model

Because the AMC adopts the university's identity, there could be a conflict of interest between the AMC-SOM and the SOM, which also represents the ZJU brand. For example, the AMC-SOM could compete for students and resources with the training and research activities of the current SOM.

The main strength of the AMC-led system is that it contains the organizational structure that facilitates many of the attributes that we have identified as keys to a successful AMC. These include (1) establishment of the university's identity as the AMC's identity, (2) a shared governance and operations control system, and (3) the pooling of financial resources and centralized management of finances under the guidance of the AMC-SOM.

However, the AMC's independence from the rest of the university will make it challenging to translate this structure to the ZJU Medical System, and there are risks that it could face conflicts of interest with the rest of the system. As such, the main value of the AMC-led system is as a pilot to demonstrate the feasibility of integration for a larger university-wide effort at a later date. At the same time, however, if the AMC-led system is a success, efforts to later integrate it into a university-wide system may be resisted by the AMC management.

Hospital-led Model

Under this system, one of the affiliated hospitals is designated as the entity responsible for establishing the AMC. The hospital provides the AMC with its identity and is responsible for managing AMC operations. This model most closely resembles Charite–Berlin University's hospital. Although Charite-Berlin did not form a part of our case studies and it is not a model we analyzed in Chapter Four, this model was studied by ZJU management, which provided extensive information to us for use in this report.

Ownership and Identity

Under such a system, the AMC is a unit owned partly by the university (research and training) and partly by a hospital (clinical care functions). The AMC adopts the identity of the hospital. In the case of ZJU's AMC, given the status of land ownership at the AMC and existing arrangements, First Affiliated Hospital would be a likely candidate for the lead entity were this model to be selected.

Governance and Operations

Governance is shared between the hospital and the university. The hospital operates the AMC and will appoint its leadership, including the CEO. AMC leadership reports to a board of trustees appointed by and reporting to the hospital president. The board of trustees would include representation from the affiliated hospitals, in addition to the SOM.

The AMC would enter into contractual relations with the SOM and other affiliated hospitals for linkages in recruitment, training, research, and care. The AMC staff are employees of the hospital.

The AMC would establish an AMC-H and an AMC-SOM.

The AMC would adopt the organizational structure of the parent hospital. Typically, this would include vice president–level appointees for research, education, and clinical care, in addition to administrative leadership.

The AMC under guidance from the hospital would decide on the allocation of employee time, salaries, and promotion decisions, in consultation with the employee and academic divisions and the AMC-H.

Finances

The AMC-H generates revenues primarily from clinical care and professional consultation. Fees generated from clinical services largely fund clinical care. Student fees and research grants fund the AMC SOM's core activities.

The AMC-H and AMC-SOM pool net revenues, after meeting the clinical care costs of the AMC-H and the costs of training and research of the AMC-SOM. The hospital's board of trustees is responsible for meeting deficits and allocating surpluses. However, it is important to note that clinical care could be prioritized over research and training in a hospital-led system. Resources for the latter two might be unstable as a result.

Establishment

Establishment of a hospital-led AMC system could be straightforward for clinical care activities, because these are already part of the lead hospital's activities. The lead hospital would continue with its core activities and would add management of the AMC to its tasks.

It would be costlier to establish the activities of the AMC-SOM, as this would be a new activity for the lead hospital. As noted above, the ZJU SOM could provide support for this. The other affiliated hospitals could also provide support to fill gaps in clinical care and clinical research activities.

Strengths and Weaknesses of the Model

One of the concerns about this model is whether the lead hospital will initially have the capacity to manage the AMC-SOM. To address this, the AMC may enter into an agreement with the existing SOM of the university to assist with the establishment of the system.

This model faces the disadvantages of the absence of a clear linkage with ZJU's identity and that of the AMC, whose primary identity will be that of the hospital. This could lead to a reduction in staff commitment within the AMC, as well as low commitment from the ZJU SOM and the other hospitals.

The main advantage of the hospital-led AMC is that, due to its unified governance under the hospital's leadership, there is likely to be a high level of integration between the clinical care activities of the AMC and its other activities, such as research and training. The pooling of financial resources would help ensure the financial stability of the system, as it would address the problem of the SOM being a net user of funds and the hospital being a net generator of funds.

For the lead hospital, the AMC is an extension and potential enhancement of its identity. For the SOM, however, an improved identity for the AMC could create a conflict with its own identity. Other affiliated hospitals could also face the same conflicts of interest and might need further incentivization in order to fully participate in the AMC.

The AMC governance system could also prioritize the activities of its managing entity (the hospital) over the activities of the rest of the system. This could lead to a neglect of the education and research activities, particularly in the training of MS and Ph.D. students and basic science research. It could also lead to the neglect of the interests of the other hospitals in leveraging the AMC to improve their activities. Thus, it could have limited benefits for the rest of the ZJU Medical System.

Shared Model

Under this system, the university designates one of the hospitals (the "lead hospital") to work with the SOM in a shared governance model. The AMC's features (ownership, identity, governance and operations, and finances) are hybrids that derive from one or the other of the governing entities. Of the AMCs we studied, Harvard University most closely resembles this model, although its affiliated hospitals adopt multiple identities depending on their needs, as discussed earlier.

Ownership and Identity
Under this model, the hospital and the existing SOM would jointly create and govern the new AMC. Note that the hospital and SOM own and operate their own physical assets, such as infrastructure, and employ their own human resources. They would allocate resources to the AMC to develop infrastructure and add employees. Therefore, under this system, the employees of the AMC would belong to either the hospital or the SOM.

Under the agreement to create the AMC, the university imparts its identity to the AMC.

Governance and Operations

The hospital and SOM share governance of the AMC. The executive leadership of the AMC, including the CEO of the AMC, is appointed by and reports to a board of trustees consisting of representatives of the hospital and the SOM.

The AMC's training functions would be owned and operated by the SOM. The AMC's clinical care functions would be owned and operated by the hospital. Research ownership and operation would vary by type. The SOM would own and operate basic science, translational, and interdisciplinary research, and the hospital would own and operate clinical research.

Unlike the AMC-led and hospital-led models, there is no need for separate divisions, such as the AMC-SOM and AMC-H, because of the shared ownership and governance structure.

Finances

The hospital generates revenue from clinical care. Clinical care is largely funded by health insurance. Clinical research is funded both by hospital revenues and external sources of funding, such as government grants.

Student fees, university support, and research grants fund the SOM's core activities.

The SOM's core activities, training, and research benefit the hospital through improved brand recognition, higher-quality faculty, and other long-term benefits.

The hospital pays an annual fee to the university in return for these long-term benefits and to support research or student training. To ensure financial stability of the AMC, the fees could be paid as part of a long-term arrangement between the hospital and the AMC.

Establishment

For the most part, establishment of a shared operation system is relatively low cost and quick. This is because the expertise for the different activities already exists in other parts of the ZJU system and could be transferred by the SOM and the lead hospital. Creating the envisaged structure would primarily require creating the coordinating positions and initiatives described earlier.

Strengths and Weaknesses of the Model

This model promotes a common ZJU identity. This factor and the ease of establishment are the main strengths. However, it is likely to face considerable challenges. The model assumes that the hospitals will gain something from engaging with the SOM. Currently, there is little incentive for the hospitals to subsume their identity to the university.[2] Among the consequences of this model could be a reduction in staff commitment and low functional integration of the research functions and the care-research linkages. Therefore, the ZJU AMC would need to identify some "carrots" to entice the hospitals to engage with the SOM, employ resources in building a common brand identity through hires and conferences, or some combination thereof. These options would entail time and cost.

This model mimics, to an extent, the existing system at ZJU. The absence of a system to direct resources across the system means that the AMC will face some of the same challenges as ZJU currently faces in financial stability, such as inadequacy of resources for training and research. There could be limited effects on the rest of the ZJU Medical System.

University-Led Model

Under this system, ownership is divided between the university and the hospital, and governance is shared between the university and the hospital. The AMC adopts the identity of the university and is operated by the university.

Stanford and UCLA are most similar to this model, although they exhibit many features of the shared governance model as well. UW also shares features of this model.

Ownership and Identity
Under such a system, the AMC is a unit owned partly by the university (research and training) and partly by a hospital (clinical care functions). The AMC adopts the university's identity.

Governance and Operations
Governance is shared between the hospital and the university. The SOM operates the AMC and appoints its leadership, including the CEO. It enters into contractual relations with the other affiliated hospitals for linkages in recruitment, training, research, and care.

All AMC employees, including all hospital staff and SOM staff, are employees of the university.

The university designates the SOM as the lead entity for governing the AMC and appointing its leadership. The AMC leadership reports to a board of trustees appointed by and reporting to the SOM dean. AMC leadership should include representation from the affiliated hospitals, in addition to the SOM.

---

2   It should be noted that mere physical proximity will not encourage integration, commitment to a single identity, and equitable resource allocation. This is why coordinating positions are needed to help facilitate these relationships.

The AMC creates separate divisions for training and research within the AMC-SOM and clinical care within the AMC-H. The AMC-SOM's core activities are training and oversight of all research. The AMC-H's core activity is clinical care.

The AMC's training functions and all research are operated by the AMC under guidance from the SOM. The SOM also provides staffing support to the AMC. One or more affiliated hospitals under contract provide the AMC's clinical care functions.

The AMC, under guidance from its board of trustees, decides on the allocation of employee time, salaries, and promotion decisions in consultation with the employee and academic divisions and the AMC-H.

Finances

The AMC-H generates revenues from clinical care. Health insurance largely funds clinical care. Student fees, university support, and research grants fund the AMC-SOM's core activities of training and research. The AMC-H and AMC-SOM pool net revenues, after meeting clinical care costs of the AMC-H and costs of training and research of the AMC-SOM. Deficits, if any, are funded by transfers from the university.

Establishment

Establishment of this model is likely to be simpler than the AMC-led system, because the expertise to run the training and basic research activities already resides within the SOM. Adding the clinical care and research activities would require building contractual relations with the hospitals, which would entail time and cost. This has the advantage of tapping different hospitals' resources, as opposed to relying on a single hospital.

Strengths and Weaknesses of the Model

Because the AMC is directly governed by the SOM, the SOM would not face any conflicts of interest with the AMC. Instead, the SOM would view the AMC as a way to enhance its brand through better integration of its own training and research functions with the other components of the ZJU Medical System.

The shared operational system could also work to the advantage of the hospitals. For the affiliated hospitals, the AMC could facilitate the strengthening of the hospitals' clinical research capacities by enabling the best physician-researchers from the hospitals to spend time at the AMC. The AMC could also be a venue for specialists at different affiliated hospitals to work together on both research and care. Because the hospitals already have their own identities, they would not face conflicts of interest arising from identity issues.

The system of unifying all research operations under the SOM is expected to promote functional integration of the different research activities. The main strength of the university-led system, like the AMC-led system, is that it contains the organizational structure that facilitates many of the attributes that we have identified as being key to a successful AMC. These include (1) the establishment of the university's identity as its identity, (2) a shared governance and operations control system, and (3) the pooling of financial resources and centralized management of finances under the guidance of the AMC-SOM. Hence, it potentially achieves many of the attributes that we have identified as key attributes for the ZJU AMC. These include staff commitment, leveraging the ZJU identity, promoting functional integration, and promoting internal interaction and external collaborations.

Due to its unified management of financial resources, this system is well-positioned to address the problem of the SOM being a net user of funds and the hospital being a net generator of funds, thus helping the AMC achieve financial stability while allocating resources fairly across all entities.

Furthermore, unlike the AMC-led system, the university-led system has the advantage of integration with the university and its affiliated hospitals right from the start because of the absence of conflicts of interest.

Summary of the Models

Table 5.1 summarizes the differences between the organizational domains across the different models. It also provides information on the relative costs and times to establishment between the different models.

Table 5.1
Organizational Options Summary

Model	Organizational Domains			
	Ownership and Identity	**Governance and Operations**	**Finances**	**Establishment**
AMC-led	• AMC is owned by the university and the hospital. It adopts the identity of the university.	• University appoints AMC's BOT. • BOT includes representation of SOM and hospitals. • AMC operates independently of other entities. • AMC establishes hospital, SOM and research divisions for care, research, and training, respectively. • Physical assets, such as infrastructure, and employees belong to the university.	• Hospital and SOM division's net revenues are pooled. • AMC uses the surplus for long-term developmental initiatives.	• Establishment requires collaboration with existing hospitals and the SOM and takes time and resources. • Establishment and integration into the university-wide health system could face capacity constraints.

Table 5.1—Continued

Model	Organizational Domains			
	Ownership and Identity	Governance and Operations	Finances	Establishment
Hospital-led	• AMC is owned by the university and the hospital. It adopts the identity of the hospital.	• Hospital appoints the AMC's BOT. • BOT includes representation of SOM and hospitals. • AMC establishes hospital and SOM divisions for care (AMC-H), training, and research (AMC-SOM). • All the physical assets, such as infrastructure and employees, belong to the hospital.	• Hospital and SOM net revenues are pooled. • Hospital allocates surplus and meets deficit.	• Establishment of the hospital division is relatively quick and low cost. • Establishment of the SOM division takes time and resources.
Shared	• AMC adopts the identity of the university. • The hospital owns the clinical care and research functions of the AMC, including the physical infrastructure and employees. • The SOM owns the training and nonclinical research functions of the AMC, including the physical infrastructure and employees.	• The university appoints the BOT, which includes representatives of the hospitals and the SOM. • The university designates one the of the hospitals as the lead hospital.	• The hospital and SOM manage their own revenues and costs. • Hospital pays into a fund to support research and training with a pre-agreed share of the hospital's revenues.	• Establishment is relatively low cost and quick.

Table 5.1—Continued

	Organizational Domains			
Model	**Ownership and Identity**	**Governance and Operations**	**Finances**	**Establishment**
University-led	• AMC is owned by the university and the hospital. It adopts the identity of the university. • All the physical assets, such as infrastructure and employees, belong to the university.	• SOM appoints the AMC's BOT and the AMC leadership. • BOT includes representation of SOM and hospitals. • AMC establishes divisions for care (AMC-H), and training and research (AMC-SOM).	• Hospital and SOM net revenues are pooled. • AMC uses the surplus for long-term developmental initiatives.	• Establishment of the SOM division is faster and less costly than the AMC-led system. • Establishment of the hospital division requires new arrangements with existing hospitals to support clinical care at the AMC and is time-consuming and costly.

BOT = Board of Trustees.

Table 5.2, which is the analog to Table 3.1, maps the entities that are the main drivers of operational activities under different AMC models.

The analysis regarding the strengths and weaknesses of the different models is summarized in Table 5.3. To highlight performance, we have shaded desirable traits in green and less desirable traits in red.

Table 5.3 suggests that two models appear to best address the challenges. The university-led system positively affects the most desired attributes both within the AMC and the rest of the system. The AMC-led system positively affects most desired attributes within the AMC but not outside of it. Accordingly, we recommend that the university-led system be adopted. If that is not immediately feasible, then the AMC-led system should be considered as a starting point, with a commitment and plan to move to the university-led system over time.

Table 5.2
Entities Mapped to Operations in the AMC Models

Operational Activities	Model			
	AMC-led	Hospital-led	Shared	University-led
Clinical research	Research division	Hospital	Hospital	SOM
Basic science, interdisciplinary, and translational research	Research division	Hospital	SOM	SOM
Training MDs	SOM division	Pre-clinical: SOM division Clinical: hospital division	SOM	SOM
Training MSs and Ph.D.s	SOM division	SOM division	SOM	SOM
Clinical care	Hospital division	Hospital	Hospital	Recruitment, allocation, and evaluation: SOM Monitoring: hospital
External collaboration	AMC	Hospital	Shared	SOM

Table 5.3
Models' Influence on Attributes

Attribute	AMC-led		Hospital-led		Shared Operations		University-led	
	Within AMC	University-wide	Within AMC	University-wide	Within AMC	University-wide	Within AMC	University-wide
Commits faculty, physicians, and affiliated entities to all activities of the AMC	Yes	No	No	No	No	No	Yes	Yes
Leverages ZJU identity	Yes	No	No	No	Yes	Yes	Yes	Yes
Governance and Operations								
Integration of basic science, clinical, and translational research	Yes	No	No	No	No	No	Yes	Yes
Integration of care and research	Yes	No	Yes	No	No	No	Yes	Yes
Integration of training and research	Yes	No	No	No	Yes	No	Yes	Yes
Integration of care and training	Yes	No	Yes	No	Yes	No	Yes	Yes
Promotes interactions within ZJU	N/A	No	N/A	No	N/A	No	N/A	Yes
Promotes external collaboration	Yes	No	No	No	No	No	Yes	Yes

Table 5.3—Continued

	Model							
	AMC-led		Hospital-led		Shared Operations		University-led	
Attribute	Within AMC	University-wide	Within AMC	University-wide	Within AMC	University-wide	Within AMC	University-wide
Financial stability—adequacy of:								
Resources for training	Yes	No	No	No	No	No	Yes	Yes
Resources for clinical research	Yes	No	Yes	No	No	No	Yes	Yes
Resources for nonclinical research	Yes	No	No	No	No	No	Yes	Yes
Resources for clinical care	Yes	No	Yes	No	Yes	No	Yes	Yes
Financial stability—cost-efficient pathways to establishment	No	N/A	No	N/A	Yes	No	No	N/A

CHAPTER SIX

Pathways, Monitoring, and Evaluation

Deciding on a suitable organizational model for ZJU's AMC system is, in some sense, the first step in an ongoing process. Those in military and emergency response organizations often say that "no plan survives first contact with reality." More than 40 years of research on program and policy implementation suggests that much the same is true of innovations involving significant organizational changes, such as those contemplated by ZJU.[1] For instance, implementation of initiatives often reveal that there is less buy-in than expected from key partners, unexpected funding challenges, unanticipated skill deficits, and bureaucratic constraints (e.g., contracting and hiring regulations). These problems are all the more prevalent in complex systems, which involve autonomous or semiautonomous partners working in changing environments.[2]

Traditionally, design and implementation of organizational innovations have been viewed as separate, discrete steps, as is illustrated in the common saying, "Plan your work, and work your plan." Given the challenges cited above, however, there is a growing tendency to view the implementation process as an opportunity to continue learning and refining the design. Indeed, many important lessons are difficult for even the most informed, thoughtful designers to anticipate.

The specific recommendations made in Chapter Five would all require this type of thoughtful design, as well as the ability to include the mechanisms for midcourse corrections in the design. For example, UW created a coordinating committee for training. This required the appointment of a CMO and collaboration between the CMO and the dean of education. ZJU could consider creating such a body for its AMC. Over time, this body could be in charge of midcourse corrections that could be implemented in a number of ways. For example, the CMO and dean of education could implement some of their decisions through departments within their divisions (i.e., the hospital and SOM), or they could leave it to the departmental heads to coor-

---

[1] D. Fixsen, S. F. Naoom, D. A. Blase, R. M. Friedman, and F. Wallace, *Implementation Research: A Synthesis of the Literature*, Tampa, Fla.: The National Implementation Research Network, University of South Florida, Louis de la Parte Florida Mental Health Institute, 2005.

[2] E. Olson and G. Eoyang, *Facilitating Organizational Change: Lessons from Complexity Science*, Hoboken, N.J.: Pfeiffer Press, 2001.

dinate across divisions. However, they might prefer to retain some of the more critical policy issues within their domains of implementation and create task forces for each major policy challenge. For example, they could delegate training curriculum development to departmental heads, while retaining the integration of care and training within their own domains. Each approach would bring its own challenges for strategy formulation and implementation.

With this is in mind, we propose an establishment process that involves (1) ongoing engagement of key partners and stakeholders, (2) identification of key assumptions, success factors, and possible failure modes, (3) thoughtful sequencing of efforts and phased implementation, and (4) ongoing monitoring and evaluation to inform the entire process. In what follows, we provide additional detail on each of these.

Engagement of Partners and Stakeholders

If ZJU decides to proceed as recommended in this report, it should, as soon as possible, convene an internal Design and Implementation Workgroup to advise ZJU leadership on the full range of issues related to refining the approach described earlier and implementing it. This group should include a full range of key partners and stakeholders, including but not limited to senior ZJU leadership, the SOM, partner hospitals, academic departments with research interests that overlap with the goals of the AMC (e.g., engineering, data science), government, relevant local industry, and others. Apart from leadership, it would be useful to include representation of those with a proven record of collaboration across the system for training, care, and research. The Design and Implementation Workgroup would both provide useful information and insights to the process and help ensure that other stakeholders within partner organizations are brought into the process. As such, every effort should be made to select important influencers who have stature in their respective organizations and professions. In many instances, these would also be administrative leaders. However, it would also be important to recognize other individuals, such as frontline physicians, nurses, and potentially even administrative support staff, who are respected across staff categories and can identify potential pitfalls to implementation.

Identification of Key Assumptions, Success Factors, and Possible Failure Modes

In order to help ensure that the implementation effort is focused on the most important factors, there should be an early effort to articulate intermediate and ultimate outcomes—that is, to provide answers to the following three questions:

1. How will we know if the organizational model selected and implemented is working?
2. What are the factors most likely to influence success?
3. How is the model most likely to fail?

One common method to achieve this is through the creation of logic models that show visually how various resources and processes might relate to outputs and outcomes. Logic models are useful conceptually because they identify the linkages between inputs, outputs, and outcomes; the resources required for each process; and the assumptions and risks of each process.[3]

Such models are often most useful if developed through a collaborative process and could be developed with input from the Design and Implementation Workgroup. Such a model should also include outcomes of interest to identify progress toward goals. It will be important to identify long-term outcomes (e.g., overall research funding) with intermediate and even short-term outcomes (e.g., increases in the frequency and quality of multidisciplinary collaborations; collaborations between researchers and clinicians; the balance of care between comprehensive and specialized care; and innovative practices). For each, the logic modeling process could involve identifying the most important resources and processes needed and also ways in which achieving these outcomes is most likely to fail. The deliberations of the Design and Implementation Workgroup should be supplemented, where possible, with reviews of relevant literature and best practices, as well as examination of past experience at ZJU and elsewhere. For instance, Design and Implementation Workgroup members might find that past efforts at collaboration have been hindered by differences across partner institutions in contracting procedures, a lack of time for staff to devote to joint resources, or differences in professional language and culture across institutions and disciplines.

Sequencing of Efforts and Phased Implementation

With this understanding of outcomes, drivers, and failure models in hand, the Design and Implementation Workgroup can advise ZJU on the most logical sequence in which to implement its desired system, attempting to ensure that the necessary drivers are put into place early, and that there are efforts to prevent or mitigate likely failure points. For example, integrating the different research streams (basic science, translational, and clinical) may require a change in how resources have historically been committed, networks of teams created, and researchers incentivized. This is a challenge faced by leading AMCs around the world, and they have approached it in different ways. Iden-

---

[3]   Burt Perrin, *Moving from Outputs to Outcomes: Practical Advice from Governments Around the World*, Washington, D.C.: World Bank, January 2006.

tifying a pathway that is feasible, efficient, and effective will require understanding resource needs, the career goals of researchers, and revisions in organizational models. Implementing a pathway to a desired system will likely require monitoring processes and evaluating outcomes regularly and making changes as new knowledge is gained.

The Design and Implementation Workgroup and ZJU leadership might also seek to identify "early wins"—that is, steps that help demonstrate success and mutual benefit of the AMC early in the process as a way to build support and momentum for later efforts. Similarly, they could prioritize early development efforts for which there are promising funding sources, whether through philanthropies, industry, government, or others. For instance, ZJU could select, as an early priority, a search for ways to leverage the brand name of the university in all AMC operations. Attaching the ZJU brand name to every activity is not a simple exercise. It requires at least considering which activities can assume the ZJU name right away and those that are not yet ready. There could even be activities that would add value to the ZJU name. In this way, an exercise of identification will allow the AMC to quickly use the ZJU name for selected activities while using the exercise to identify areas for improvement in activities not ready for branding.

A related initiative may be to begin crafting goals for the identity of the university's AMC, because the two best models involve some degree of identity shift for several of the organizations within the AMC enterprise. It will then be necessary to determine the best ways to achieve those goals (e.g., through recruiting, conferences).

Another early initiative could be the creation of multidisciplinary Centers of Excellence that are funded by the private and public sector with a mandate to solve specific cutting-edge research problems of these sectors through multidisciplinary efforts. For example, health care equipment companies might be willing to support a Center of Excellence focused on medical device discovery or the application of artificial intelligence to providing solutions for diagnosis or monitoring.

Ongoing Monitoring and Evaluation to Inform the Entire Process

Given the likelihood of unanticipated barriers and consequences, it is important that all aspects of design and implementation be informed by ongoing monitoring and evaluation. These factors together would ensure the presence of learning and feedback loops that can guide ZJU in making midcourse corrections.

Ongoing monitoring. The logic modeling exercise described earlier could provide the basis for developing measurable indicators of key processes and outcomes, as well as factors that might anticipate deviations from key assumptions or success factors. An effort should be made to measure not only desired outcomes (e.g., funded multidisciplinary projects) but intermediate outcomes (e.g., proposals developed and submitted, joint contracting processes put into place) that can help ZJU leaders and stakeholders know whether they are on the right track. Data for such indicators could come from a combination of sources, including administrative data (e.g., proposal databases), patient charts (e.g., to determine whether concepts developed through research are implemented at the bedside), surveys (e.g., of faculty, staff and patients), and periodic interviews and focus groups (e.g., to gain a more nuanced understanding of barriers, success factors). Indeed, using a combination of qualitative and quantitative data can lend greater nuance to the findings and help direct any needed course corrections. Such monitoring efforts can be conducted either by internal ZJU staff and students, or by outside consultants and researchers. Any results should be made available to ZJU leadership, the Design and Implementation Workgroup, and other stakeholders on a regular basis.

Periodic evaluations. In addition to ongoing monitoring, it is often helpful to commission discrete evaluations that examine specific topics. At least some evaluations should be conducted by independent third parties in order to ensure objectivity and should provide a more in-depth examination of issues around causal attribution than is possible via ongoing monitoring. Data sources for such evaluations can be the same as those in use for monitoring, but they may also include data collection specific to a given evaluation study.

A coordinated approach to evaluation might involve laying out an overall evaluation plan in advance, comprising both ongoing monitoring and periodic evaluation. There are several benefits to this approach. First, certain baseline data cannot be collected retrospectively. In addition, given the number of partners in the ZJU AMC, it will be important to minimize the burdens of data collection. Having an overall evaluation plan can help ensure that data are collected efficiently and without duplicative effort. Finally, an overall evaluation plan will help ensure that needed evaluations are conducted for the topics needed covering the timelines required. Such an evaluation plan may need to be updated periodically to respond to evaluation needs not apparent upon creation of the original version. However, the process of periodically reconsidering and revising the plan where necessary can be useful to promote shared learning among key stakeholders and partners.

CHAPTER SEVEN

Conclusion

The ZJU AMC is poised to have significant and important effects on the health services of Yuhang District, the medical education of the health care workforce, and national and global research discoveries. The key goals in the creation of the ZJU AMC are to:

- Provide environments that promote the creation of knowledge and innovation. This could be achieved in various ways, such as integrating research more closely with practice and collaborative learning from within the AMC, as well from other organizations in the national and global health care environment.
- Implement high-quality solutions that are consistent with global best practices.
- Be sustainable in terms of manpower, physical infrastructure, and finances, while remaining compliant with local laws, regulations, and capacity constraints.

Based on these goals, we examined existing AMC models and determined that the university-led model would achieve the highest level of performance on attributes that measure progress toward the ZJU AMC goals. These attributes were laid out in Table 2.1 in Chapter Two. They include commitment of all staff and affiliated entities to the activities of the AMC; leveraging of the ZJU identity; functional integration of research, care, and training; and financial stability.

A second model, the AMC-led model, also achieves the desirable attributes of the university-led system but primarily within the AMC. This model does not achieve desirable university-wide effects. However, it may be seen as a pathway to a university-led system, if so desired by ZJU leadership.

Both models entail significant start-up costs and time commitments compared with some of the other models considered. They also entail a certain organizational vision that recognizes that ownership may be separated from governance, which in turn may be separated from operations control—that is, these three aspects of the organizations may be under different entities in order to create an institution with powerful effects. A key aspect of this organizational vision is the importance of a unified identity: the university.

The case studies highlighted the role of government and private donors in enabling the success of AMCs. The role of the government will be necessary at different levels—provincial, municipal, and district. Government support is needed to ensure that establishment costs are met and to help set the vision of creating a unified health system under the identity of the university.

The process does not end with selecting a model and implementing it. There are always unanticipated challenges and unintended consequences in the process of transition. In some cases, these challenges and consequences will require "circling the wagons," and ZJU and AMC leadership will need to bring others on board with the vision and mission of the new AMC. In other cases, these challenges and consequences will indicate a need to adjust the model and the implementation planning process.

Understanding which approach is needed will require ongoing monitoring and measurement throughout the implementation process. These activities should be systematic, utilize different types of data (e.g., quantitative and qualitative) and data sources, and focus on long-term goals (e.g., sustainability) and short- and mid-term goals (e.g., number of grant applications; number of faculty retained after the first two years). Such monitoring and measurement are key to the success of the ZJU AMC, and they should be initiated in parallel with the initiation of plans for implementation of the new model.

Models of Organizational Structure

An organization responds to the goals set for it by its owners through a control system that directs resources appropriately. The organizational system consists of three tiers: the owners, a governance system, and an operations system. For a non-profit organization, the governance system is usually implemented by a board of trustees. The operations system is implemented by the management of the institution. The governing board and management have responsibilities, as follows:

Governance responsibilities:

- *Ownership:* Responsibility for maintaining legal ownership, on behalf of the owners of the institution.
- *Identity:* Responsibility for pursuing the vision and mission of the institution, and maintaining the image and brand presented to both internal and external stakeholders.
- *Setting policies:* Identify the broad (systemwide) results to be achieved by the organization.

Operational responsibilities:

- *Determining outcomes:* The specific, measurable results to be achieved by the organization in order to fulfill the desired identity and policy priorities.
- *Determining strategy:* A description of how an outcome will be achieved through the specification of action plans and resource requirements.
- *Determining and implementing the action plan:* A sequence of steps that must be taken or tasks or activities that must be performed to achieve the strategy.
- *Resource management:* Acquisition and deployment of staff, tangible assets, intangible assets (e.g., licenses), and operating items necessary to implement, monitor, and evaluate action plans.

Figure A.1 summarizes the relationship between the above components.

Figure A.1
The Relationship Between Ownership, Identity, Governance, and Operations

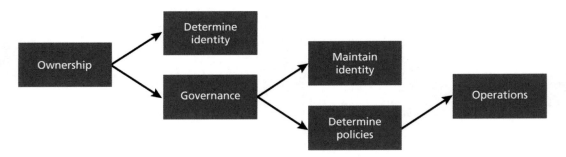

To determine the appropriate control system for the ZJU AMC, we considered various possibilities. Table A.1 lists these possibilities; Table A.2 shows the operational control in the case studies we examined.

In the case of the ZJU AMC, ownership is divided. This suggests that a shared governance structure may be appropriate. Our case studies show that shared governance is selected even when ownership belongs to single entity. This suggests the following feasible combinations (see Table A.3) for the ZJU AMC.

Table A.3 presents six possible combinations. Reviewing these against the desired attributes of the AMC presented in Chapter Two, we note that leveraging the ZJU identity is a key attribute desired by the ZJU Medical System. Hence, we exclude from further consideration the following two cases: O_d, G_s, I_h, F_a and O_d, G_s, I_h, F_s. This leaves four cases, which we considered further in Chapter Four.

Table A.1
Tiers of Organizational Control

Ownership[a]	Governance[b]	Identity[c]	Operational Control[d]
University	University	University	University
Hospital	Hospital	Hospital	Hospital
Divided	Shared		Autonomous
			Shared

[a] Ownership: There are two possible owners of the AMC, the university and the hospital. The university and hospital may not be independently owned and instead may have an ownership relationship. For example, the university may own the hospital in full or part, or vice versa. For our purposes, we assume, regardless of the ownership relationship between the university and the hospital, that they are governed and operate autonomously of each other. Ownership of the AMC may lie with either the university or the hospital or may be divided between them.

[b] Governance: *Governance* derives from ownership. This assumes, in case ownership is by a single entity, that the owner will always have a role in governance, but may share that role with another entity. By sharing, we mean that governance may either be jointly exercised or divided in an agreed way. If ownership is divided, governance will always be shared.

[c] Identity: *Identity* derives from governance and is unique, not shared. In the event of shared governance, the governing board determines which identity to impart to the AMC.

[d] Operational Control: *Operational control* derives from governance and identity. This assumes that operational control may not lie solely with an entity that is not part of the governance system and not part of the identity. However, operational control may always be shared or autonomously exercised.

Table A.2
Organizational Control of Case Studies

Case Studies	Ownership (O)	Governance (G)	Identity (I)	Operational Control (F)	Organizational System
UW	University	Shared	University	University	O_u, G_s, I_u, F_u
Stanford University, UCLA	University	Shared	University	Shared	O_u, G_s, I_u, F_s
Charite-Berlin	Hospital	Hospital	Hospital	Hospital	O_h, G_h, I_h, F_h
Harvard University	Divided	Shared	University	Shared	O_d, G_s, I_u, F_s

NOTE: In the "Organizational System" column, uppercase letters O, G, I, and F refer to "Ownership," "Governance," "Identity," and "Operational Control," respectively. The subscript letters refer to the types within the tiers of control; a = autonomous, h = hospital, s = shared, u = university.

Table A.3
Models of Organizational Control

Ownership (O)	Governance (G)	Identity (I)	Operational Control (F)	Feasible Organizational Models	System
Divided	Shared	University	University	O_d, G_s, I_u, F_u	University-led
		Hospital	Hospital	O_d, G_s, I_u, F_a	AMC-led
			Autonomous	O_d, G_s, I_u, F_s	Shared
			Shared	O_d, G_s, I_h, F_h	Hospital-led
				O_d, G_s, I_h, F_a	AMC-led
				O_d, G_s, I_h, F_s	Shared

NOTE: Ownership status is divided. The ZJU AMC consists of a hospital, owned by First Affiliated Hospital, which is one of the eight hospitals affiliated with ZJU; and a research wing, owned by the university. As noted earlier, because ownership is divided, governance will be shared. Combinations O_d, G_s, I_u, F_h and O_d, G_s, I_h, F_u are omitted based on the argument as noted in Table A.1 (i.e., that operational control may not lie solely with an entity that is not part of the governance system and not part of the identity). In the "Feasible Organizational System" column, uppercase letters O, G, I, and F refer to "Ownership," "Governance," "Identity," and "Operational Control," respectively. The subscript letters refer to the types within the tiers of control; a = autonomous, h = hospital, s = shared, u = university.

Case Study Selection

We identified the four AMCs for case studies using the following procedure:

1. For reasons of manageability, we restricted the list to SOMs based in the United States. Given that ZJU is a public university, we decided to include at least two public universities in the final list. Furthermore, the selected schools needed to be organized as AMCs rather than stand-alone SOMs.
2. Using a well-regarded university-ranking system, the QS World University Rankings,[1] we listed those in the global top 25 that are based in the United States. Twelve U.S. schools made the list. These were, in order of rank:
   a. Harvard University
   b. Stanford University
   c. Johns Hopkins University
   d. UCLA
   e. Yale University
   f. Massachusetts Institute of Technology
   g. University of California, San Francisco
   h. Columbia University
   i. University of Pennsylvania
   j. University of California, San Diego
   k. Duke University
   l. UW.
3. Harvard University and Stanford University were short-listed for their No. 1 and No. 2 rankings.
4. UCLA was short-listed for being the highest-ranking public university.
5. Because the next several public universities were also from the University of California system, we decided to exclude them due to concerns that they might have similar organizational structures.

---

[1] The medical schools of Harvard University, Stanford University, UCLA, and UW were ranked No. 1, No. 4, No. 7 and No. 24, respectively, in the world in 2018 by QS Top Universities (see QS, "QS World University Rankings: Medicine," webpage, undated.

6. UW, as the next–highest-ranking public university, was chosen to be the fourth on our short list.

7. All four schools in the short list are organized as AMCs. We talked to contacts at each site to ensure that there was enough variation in organizational domains within the group to derive useful conclusions. The list also met some key client aspirations: high global ranking (all); leadership in innovation including in medical technology (all, but particularly Stanford); leadership in accessing public funds for research within the public university setting (UW); and, again, within a public university setting, apparent success with integrating an initially autonomous SOM and hospital into an integrated AMC (UCLA).

8. We reviewed the short list with the client before final selection.

References

Association of Academic Health Centers, "Academic Health Centers: Leading Healthcare Transformation," webpage, undated. As of October 15, 2018:
http://www.aahcdc.org/21st-Century-AHCs/
Academic-Health-Centers-Leading-Healthcare-Transformation

Australian Government, Department of Education and Training, "Implementation Measures Released for China's New-World Class University Policy," January 2017. As of October 15, 2018:
https://internationaleducation.gov.au/News/Latest-News/Pages/Implementation-measures-released-for-China%E2%80%99s-new-world-class-university-policy.aspx

Barnard, Chester I., and Kenneth R. Andrews, *The Functions of the Executive*, Vol. 11, Cambridge, Mass.: Harvard University Press, 1968.

Barney, Jay B., "Organizational Culture: Can It Be a Source of Sustained Competitive Advantage?" *Academy of Management Review*, Vol. 11, No. 3, 1986, pp. 656–665.

Blakely, C., J. Meyer, R. Gottschalk, N. Schmidt, W. Davidson, D. Roitman, and J. Emshoff, "The Fidelity-Adaptation Debate: Implications for the Implementation of Public Sector Social Programs," *American Journal of Community Psychology*, Vol. 15, No. 3, 1987, pp. 253–268.

Bodily, Susan J., Thomas K. Glennan, Jr., Kerri A. Kerr, and Jolene R. Galegher, "Introduction: Framing the Problem," in Thomas K. Glennan, Jr., Susan J. Bodily, Jolene Galegher, and Kerri A. Kerr, *Expanding the Reach of Education Reforms: Perspectives from Leaders in the Scale-Up of Educational Interventions*, Santa Monica, Calif.: RAND Corporation, MG-248-FF, 2004, pp. 1–40. As of July 31, 2013:
http://www.rand.org/pubs/monographs/MG248.html

Bryson, John M., *Strategic Planning for Public and Nonprofit Organizations: A Guide to Strengthening and Sustaining Organizational Achievement*, Hoboken, N.J.: John Wiley and Sons, 2011.

Fixsen, D., S. F. Naoom, D. A. Blase, R. M. Friedman, and F. Wallace, *Implementation Research: A Synthesis of the Literature*, Tampa, Fla.: National Implementation Research Network, University of South Florida, Louis de la Parte Florida Mental Health Institute, 2005.

Greenfield, Victoria, Valerie L. Williams, and Elisa Eiseman, *Using Logic Models for Strategic Planning and Evaluation: Application to the National Center for Injury Prevention and Control*, Santa Monica, Calif.: RAND Corporation, TR-370-NCIPC, 2006. As of November 13, 2018:
https://www.rand.org/pubs/technical_reports/TR370.html

Harvard Medical School, "HMS Affiliates," webpage, undated. As of October 15, 2018:
https://hms.harvard.edu/about-hms/hms-affiliates

Hoegl, Martin, Michael Gibbert, and David Mazursky, "Financial Constraints in Innovation Projects: When Is Less More?" *Research Policy*, Vol. 37, No. 8, September 2008, pp. 1382–1391.

Kezar, Adrianna, and Peter D. Eckel, "Meeting Today's Governance Challenges: A Synthesis of the Literature and Examination of a Future Agenda for Scholarship," *Journal of Higher Education*, Vol. 75, No. 4, July–August 2004, pp. 371–399.

Kurtz, M. J., and A. Schrank, "Growth and Governance: Models, Measures, and Mechanisms," *Journal of Politics*, Vol. 69, No. 2, May 2007, pp. 538–554.

Matland, Richard E., "Synthesizing the Implementation Literature: The Ambiguity-Conflict Model of Policy Implementation," *Journal of Public Administration Research and Theory: J-PART*, Vol. 5, No. 2, April 1995, pp. 145–174.

Mosse, Roberto, and Leigh Ellen Sontheimer, *Performance Monitoring Indicators Handbook (English)*, Washington, D.C.: World Bank, Technical Paper No. 334, 1996. As of November 28, 2018: http://documents.worldbank.org/curated/en/467601468739574415/ Performance-monitoring-indicators-handbook

Olson, E., and G. Eoyang, *Facilitating Organizational Change: Lessons from Complexity Science*, Hoboken, N.J.: Pfeiffer Press, 2001.

Perrin, Burt, *Moving from Outputs to Outcomes: Practical Advice from Governments Around the World*, Washington, D.C.: World Bank, January 2006. As of November 28, 2018: http://siteresources.worldbank.org/CDFINTRANET/Resources/PerrinReport.pdf

Pugh, D.S., *Organization Theory: Selected Readings*, Vol. 126, Harmondsworth, UK: Penguin, 1971.

QS Top Universities, "QS World University Rankings: Medicine," webpage, undated. As of October 15, 2018: https://www.topuniversities.com/university-rankings/university-subject-rankings/2018/medicine

Vrotsos, Luke W., "White Coats Face Red Balance Sheets at Harvard Medical School," *Harvard Crimson*, May 23, 2018. As of October 15, 2018: https://www.thecrimson.com/article/2018/5/23/yir-hms-financial-woes/

Wegner, Gregory R., "Academic Health Center Governance and the Responsibilities of University Boards and Chief Executives (Report of a Symposium)," Washington, D.C.: Association of Governing Boards of Universities and Colleges, Occasional Paper 50, 2003. As of October 15, 2018: https://eric.ed.gov/?id=ED482376